Stress

The Psychology of Managing Pressure

How to turn Pressure into Positive Energy In 5 Simple Steps

Antony Felix

Your Free Gift

As a way of thanking you for the purchase, I'd like to offer you a complimentary gift:

- **5 Pillar Life Transformation Checklist:** This short book is about life transformation, presented in bit size pieces for easy implementation. I believe that without such a checklist, you are likely to have a hard time implementing anything in this book and any other thing you set out to do religiously and sticking to it for the long haul. It doesn't matter whether your goals relate to weight loss, relationships, personal finance, investing, personal development, improving communication in your family, your overall health, finances, improving your sex life, resolving issues in your relationship, fighting PMS successfully, investing, running a successful business, traveling etc. With a checklist like this one, you can bet that anything you do will seem a lot easier to implement until the end. Therefore, even if you don't continue reading this book, at least read the one thing that will help you in every other aspect of your life. Grab your copy now by clicking/tapping here or simply enter http://bit.ly/2fantonfreebie into your browser. Your life will never be the same again (if you implement what's in this book), I promise.

PS: I'd like your feedback. If you are happy with this book, please leave a review on Amazon.

Introduction

Stress and its attendant psychological disorders such as depression and anxiety are some of the major causes of ailments and low productivity among the active workforce. More worrisome is the fact that despite the number of research studies conducted annually to find a lasting solution to this problem, it is still a menace in today's society.

The number of stressors we face continues to increase everyday thanks to the highly demanding nature of today's jobs and businesses. From meeting your daily targets in the workplace to running the home, several things that relate to our modern day life can scuttle your peace of mind and affect your overall mood and outlook to life. These stressors never seem to stop coming.

If you are the empathic type with an empathic nature, you even face far more stressors than the average person does because you will react emotionally to things happening around the world and to news concerning anyone you know in the same way you would react if they were issues that affect you personally.

And the sad thing is that there seems to be a direct link between stress, anxiety, and depression as all three or at least two can occur concurrently. It is easy to get into a depressed state when you feel stressed, or once depressed, be anxious.

Whichever one applies to you, this book is designed to address these three major mental conditions, help you understand what you are dealing with, and provide you with 5 key techniques that can help you overcome these problems.

Let's begin.

Table of Contents

Before we start discussing the different strategies that you can use to fight stress, anxiety and depression, it is important that you start by having an understanding of the link between the 3 mental health issues so you know what you are up against. As they say, knowing your enemy is the first step to winning any war.

Understanding the Biological Link between Stress, Anxiety & Depression

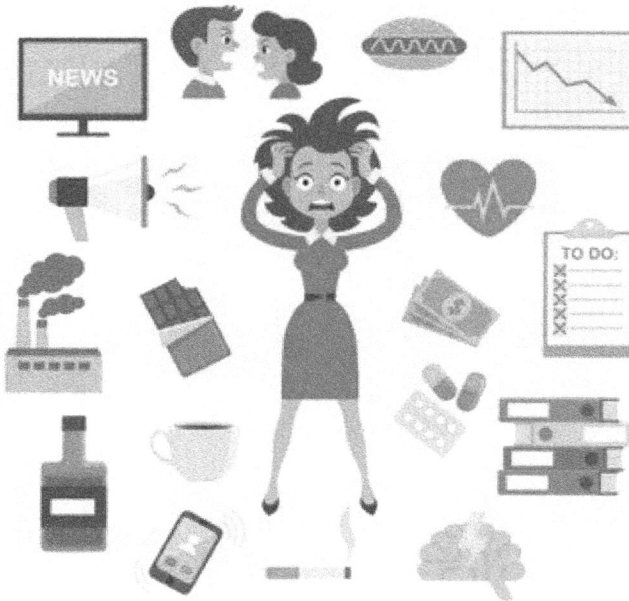

Let us understand the link between stress, anxiety, and depression before we go into techniques to beat this trio.

Researchers from the University of Ontario, Canada have this to say about the biological link between these three conditions, why one can bring about the other, and why the same techniques are effective against the three. According to Stephen Ferguson, a lead researcher at the aforementioned University, the connecting mechanism found in the human brain explains how being stressed up and anxious can make you depressed.

According to the results of the findings published online in the *Nature Neuroscience* journal, findings from this research suggest that the same drugs and treatment techniques could be selectively used to treat depressive disorders that could result from past stressful experiences.

As discovered in the research, the linking mechanism in the brain shows the interaction between the corticotrophin releasing factor receptor and certain types of serotonin receptors. The study further proved that the corticotrophin releasing factor receptor works to increase the number of serotonin receptors on cell surfaces in the human brain. This increase can lead to a level of abnormal signaling.

Since the corticotrophin receptors lead to anxiety in response to stress, and the serotonin receptors lead to depression, the research clearly shows how stress, anxiety, and depression pathways connect through very distinct processes in the human brain.

While most major depressive disorders often occur concurrently with anxiety disorders in most people, the causes for both the depression and the anxiety strongly links to very stressful experiences. In addition, there is scientific proof that stressful experiences can make the symptoms of depression and anxiety severe.

Identifying the link between these three has made it easy to choose the best treatment techniques to deal with stress and the other disorders that go along with it.

Having seen the connection between stress and its accomplices i.e. depression and anxiety, let us now see how stress affects different areas of your life.

How Stress Affects You

If there is one thing you should pay urgent attention to, it is your stress levels and the major stressors you have to deal with. Stress affects your life more than you have ever thought possible. The fact that you are not aware of the level of damage stress inflicts on you does not mean its negative effects are not as widespread as they are debilitating.

Apart from the anxiety and depressive disorders that accompany most cases of high stress levels, stress also affects your life in a number of negative ways. Below are some common ways stress affects different areas of your life and why you should deal with high stress levels as soon as possible:

Cognitive Effects of Stress

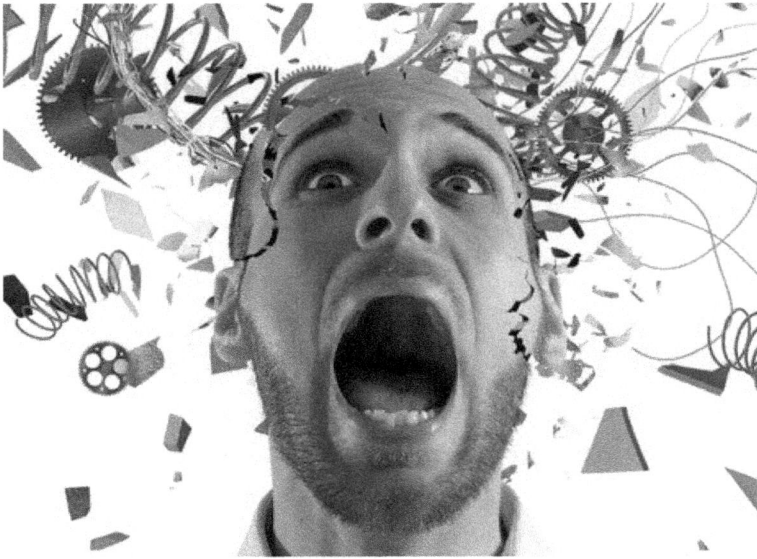

1. **Poor judgment:** High stress level has a way of clouding your sense of judgment primarily because of your inability to reason out issues objectively and intelligently.

2. **Memory problems:** People with cases of high stress levels and its attendant mental disorders also battle issues related to memory loss and inability to remember things in details.

3. **Brain fog:** One common symptom of stress most people experience is mental fatigue or confusion. This will also happen when you are either anxious or depressed. Its main characteristics are irrational thoughts running

through your mind at the same time, which leaves you fuzzy and disoriented.

4. **Lack of concentration:** It is impossible to concentrate on anything when your stress levels are at an all-time high. This is why people with high stress levels often lack motivation and the will power to get anything done.

5. **Indecision:** When you cannot concentrate because of high stress levels, it becomes increasingly difficult to make important decisions, which is why a high stress level often causes very low productivity in all areas of your life.

6. **Self-doubt:** High stress level, anxiety, and depression have a way of making you think you are not worth your salt. When you cannot seem to find your bearing, it is easy to feel inferior to others around you, which can easily lead to loss of direction.

7. **Starting several tasks and achieving very little:** In his confusion, a highly stressed person might try to get busy at several things at the same time. This is because of the confused state of mind that comes with stress. The result is dismal achievement at the end of the day.

Emotional Effects of Stress

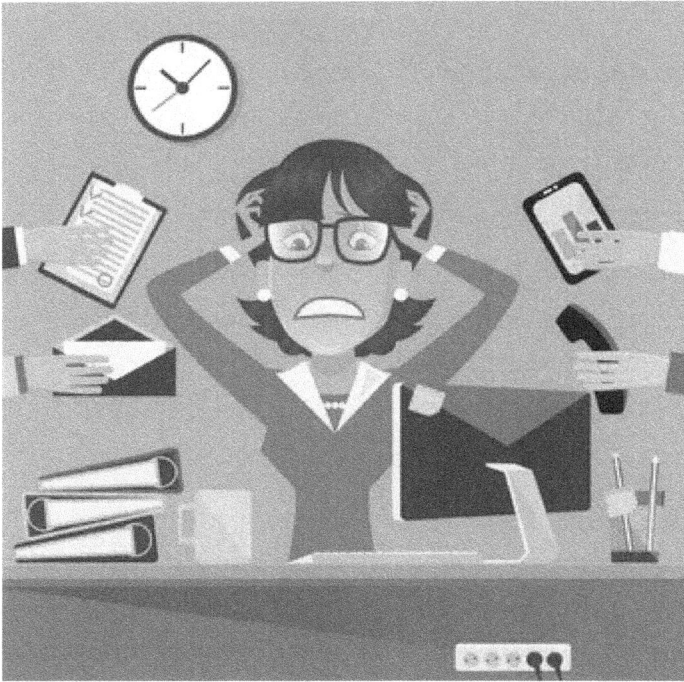

1. **Depression:** Of course, this one goes hand-in-hand with stress—as we have reiterated severally. Once your stress level stays high and unchecked for long, depression follows suit because of your inability to focus and concentrate on anything.

2. **Irritability:** Feeling easily irritated is a common adverse effect of stress. High stress levels will make you feel irritated at almost everything and everyone. This is why you see stressed people showing unexplainable anger and snapping at others at the slightest provocation.

3. **Panic:** Your high stress level will make you anxious and fearful when you have no reason to be. This is why panic disorders seem to accompany almost every case of chronic stress. Stress will keep your heart racing and skipping beats at the slightest scare.

4. **Moodiness:** A highly stressed person can be the moodiest person you can ever find anywhere. Stress comes with low spirits, lack of enthusiasm, loss of motivation and the likes, which explains why you are most likely to feel moody and unexcited when stressed out.

5. **Frustration:** Stress will make you want to give up because of frustration. This explains why people with chronic stress fall into depression easily and think suicidal thoughts.

Physical Effects of Stress

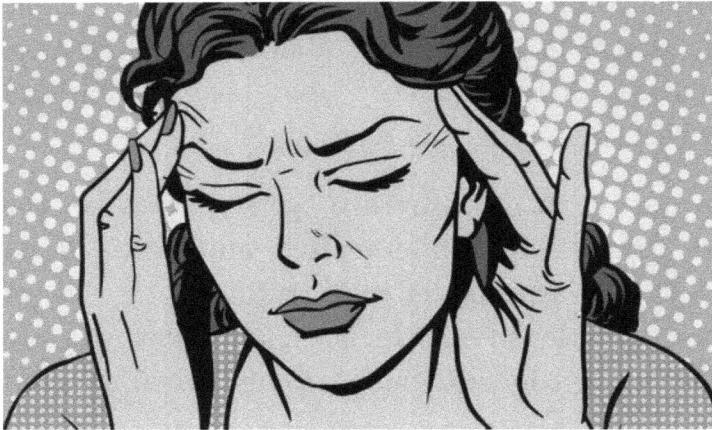

1. **Fatigues, Pains, and aches:** High stress levels will make you feel constant chest pains, aches, and fatigues. This is most common when you wake every morning after having your sleep disrupted by panic attacks and incoherent nightmares.

2. **Skin problems:** Some people with high stress level have reported an outbreak of skin problems such as acne, rashes, eczema, etc. This links back to the fact that stress affects the production of certain hormones and chemicals in the body.

3. **Indigestion:** Digestive disorders are common symptoms of stress. Stress can cause you to experience constant constipation, indigestion, and other such stomach-related problems.

4. **Rapid Heartbeat:** Your accelerated heart rate is one of the ways your body tells you it is undergoing intense pressure and needs urgent help. When such high stress levels remain unchecked for long, they can easily deteriorate into serious health problems such as high blood pressure.

Behavioral Effects of Stress

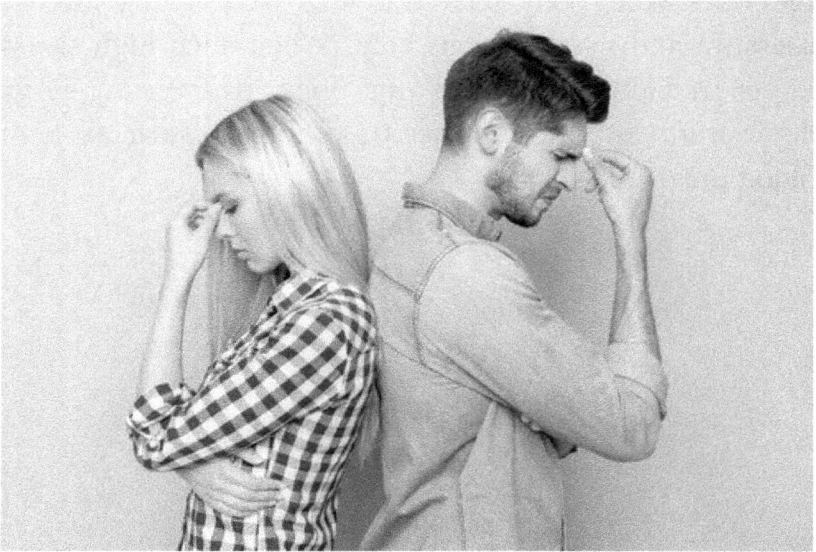

1. **Increased use of alcohol, cigarettes, and caffeine:** Stress can cause you to resort to certain unhealthy habits as a way of escape. However, most of the habits picked up as a way of dealing with stress are negative habits that end up making your situation worse. Habits such as drinking too much alcohol, smoking cigarettes, getting high on drugs and other intoxicating substances are common in people dealing with stress and depression.

2. **Lack of motivation:** Stress will take away your fighting spirit. It is hard to keep it together when stress is taking its toll on your mind and body. With a confused mind and a weak body, you can do very few things and therefore,

the earlier you deal with your stress issues, the sooner you can get your life back on track.

3. **Sleep disorders:** Stress is a known notorious sleep thief. Inadequate sleep and stress often go hand-in-hand. If you have been experiencing sleeplessness, it could be a good sign you need to pay more attention to dealing with stress.

4. **Living in isolation:** Stress will make you recline into your shell in an attempt to stay away from others who seem to be having the best time of their lives. Isolation only makes the condition worse. Hanging out with positive and fun people will do you much good.

Let us see how the stress response work and how activating the relaxation response with the right relaxation techniques can counter it and help you relax:

How the Stress Response Works

Specifically, we are going to look at the role of relaxation techniques for activating the relaxation response to counteract the natural stress response.

Relaxation Techniques

Many people assume relaxing in front of the TV is enough to make them de-stress at the end of a very stressful day. The truth remains that when it comes to beating stress, there is more to relaxation than chilling out in front of your TV set chewing your favorite popcorn.

When it comes to beating stress, you need relaxation techniques that can help you activate the relaxation response.

Relaxation Response

Whenever your stress levels get so high that your nervous system becomes overwhelmed, your body gets a boosted supply of "fight or flight" hormones. This stress response can be a real lifesaver during life-threatening emergencies where there is need for you to act very quickly. However, when the stresses of your day-to-day life and challenges constantly activate this response, it can wear you down both physically and emotionally.

While it may not be possible to avoid stress entirely, it is possible to counteract the very detrimental effects of stress by learning how to produce this all-important relaxation response, a state of deep rest considered to be the exact opposite of the stress response. This relaxation response helps bring your mind and body into the natural state of equilibrium.

Some of the things that happen when your relaxation response activates are:

1. Your muscle relax

2. Your blood pressure drops

3. Your heart rate normalizes

4. Your breathing slows down

5. Your blood flow to the brain increases.

Here, we will discuss the ability of key relaxation techniques to bring about this relaxation response; that these techniques bring about the relaxation response is what makes them ideal for fighting stress, depression, anxiety, fear and tension.

RELAXATION ROUTINE

1. SIT ON A CHAIR...

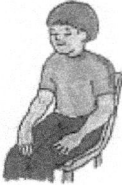

2. "SCRUNCH" UP YOUR FACE... THEN... RELAX IT...

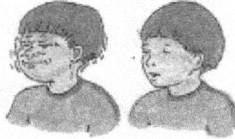

3. TENSE YOUR ARMS... THEN... RELAX THEM

4. TENSE UP YOUR SHOULDERS AND CHEST... THEN... RELAX THEM

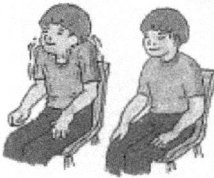

5. TENSE UP YOUR LEGS... ...THEN RELAX!

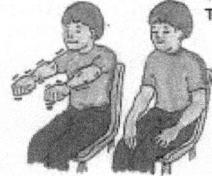

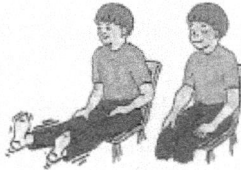

6. BREATHE IN RELAXATION... ...BREATHE OUT TENSION

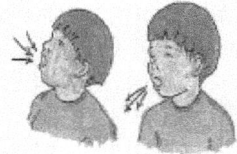

Below are the 5 key relaxation techniques you can engage in to get instant relief from stress and other mental disorders beginning with yoga:

1st Technique: Yoga Poses for Relaxation and Calmness

Yoga has the ability to combat both stress and tension effectively. In addition, regular practice, yoga will help increase your resilience when those recurring stress triggers rear up their ugly heads.

While any type of yoga is generally a good way to combat stress, we have a number of specific poses that have proven to have awesome stress-beating effects. Below are the most potent of these yoga asanas (poses):

The Eagle Pose (Garudasana)

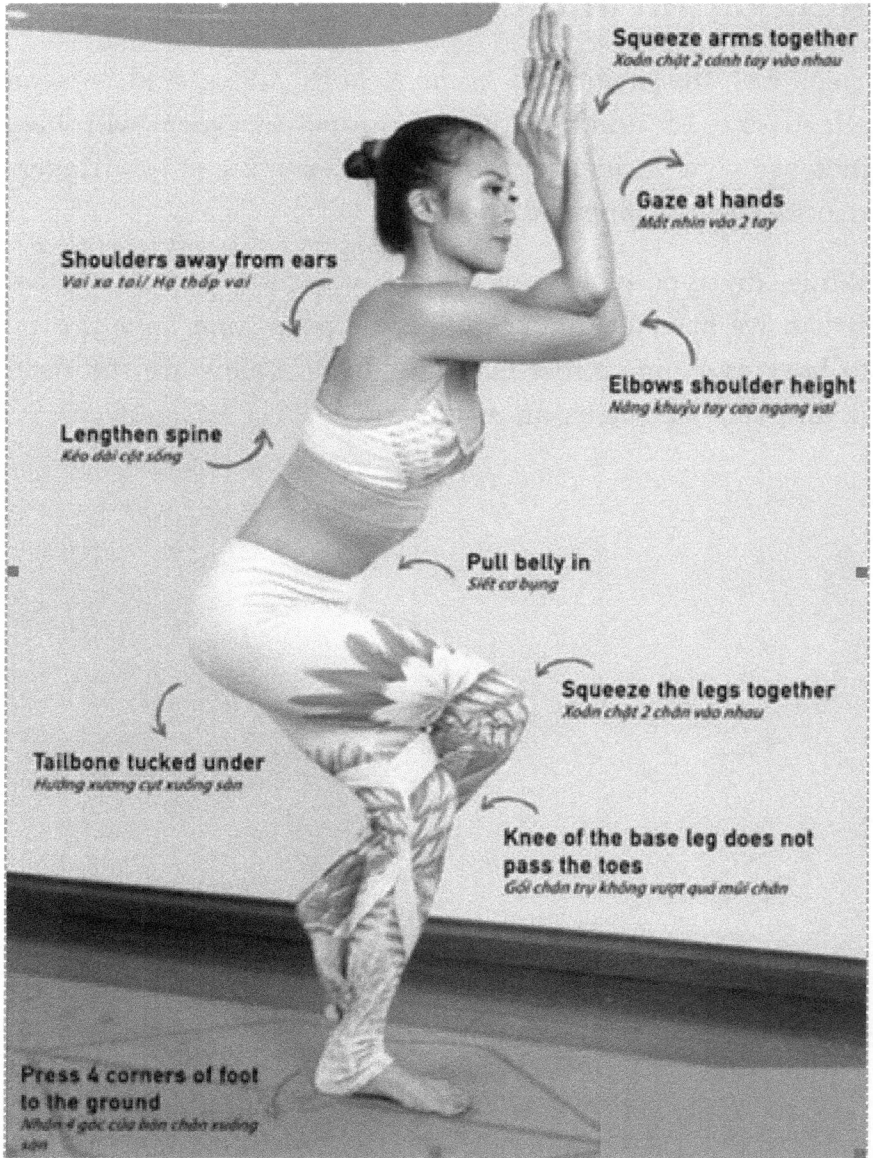

Squeeze arms together
Xoắn chặt 2 cánh tay vào nhau

Gaze at hands
Mắt nhìn vào 2 tay

Shoulders away from ears
Vai xa tai/ Hạ thấp vai

Elbows shoulder height
Nâng khuỷu tay cao ngang vai

Lengthen spine
Kéo dài cột sống

Pull belly in
Siết cơ bụng

Squeeze the legs together
Xoắn chặt 2 chân vào nhau

Tailbone tucked under
Hướng xương cụt xuống sàn

Knee of the base leg does not pass the toes
Gối chân trụ không vượt quá mũi chân

Press 4 corners of foot to the ground
Nhấn 4 góc của bàn chân xuống sàn

This yoga pose requires that you focus your mind on a single point, which is why it is a very powerful stress and tension management tool. It is also ideal for freeing up tightness around the hips and shoulders—common accumulation points for emotional stress.

Steps to the eagle pose:

1. Assume the tadasana pose (shown below), and from there, keep your feet hip-width apart while keeping your arms as widely spread as possible. Bring your right arm over your left arm.

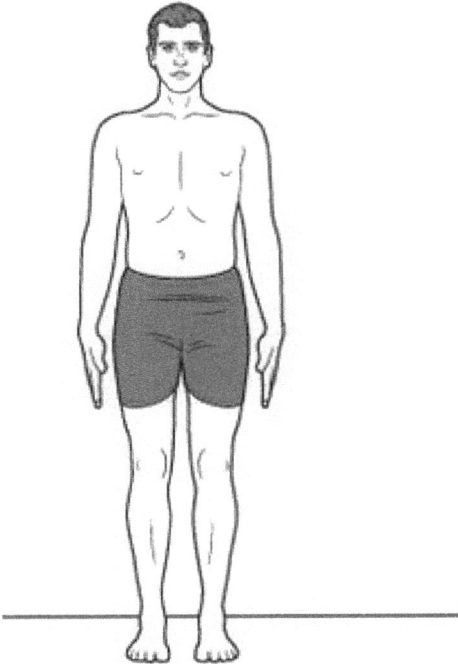

2. Then, bend your elbows and bring your palms together.

3. Shift your weight to the four corners of your right foot and bend your knees a little bit.

4. Lift your left thigh up and place it over your right thigh. If your knees feel comfortable and you are able to hook your toes behind your right calf, do so. You can leave the foot where it is if you cannot do the toe-hooking stunt. You do not have to force it: it's an anatomical feat some people can pull off naturally.

5. Engage your core and start sinking your hips down while you maintain the length of your spine. Firmly keep your gaze on the point you chose to focus on as your breath flows effortlessly.

6. To come out of this pose, begin to unwind slowly until you have returned to the Tadasana pose. You can repeat the pose on your other side.

TIP: The object you choose to fix your gaze on is an important part of the stress-relieving pose. As such, make sure you choose to focus on something that lifts your spirit naturally such as a gemstone or crystal.

The Standing Forward Fold (Uttanasana)

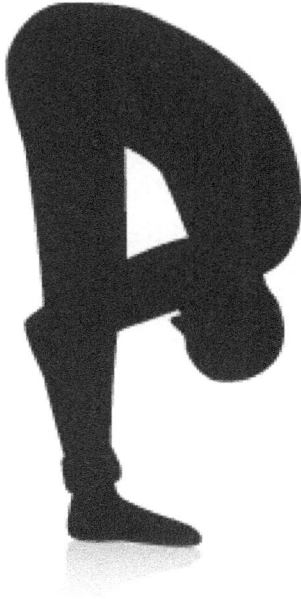

The Uttanasana pose can help you achieve a quiet and calm mind, balance your nervous system, and promote feelings of peace. It also energetically balances your sacral chakra, which when overstimulated, can contribute to excessive and fluctuating emotional energy. Uttanasana can help quiet a busy mind, balance the nervous system, and promote feelings of calm and peace.

Steps to the Uttanasana pose:

1. Start with the Tadasana pose, bend your knees, engage your core slightly, hinge forward from your hips, and then

place your hands either in front of you or alongside your feet.

2. Shift your weight to the balls of your feet and feel your sit bones lifting upwards. For very tight hamstrings, you can keep your knees bent to keep your lower back protected. Alternatively, you can lengthen through the backs of your legs as you keep your weight on the balls of your feet.

3. Take hold of each one of your elbows with your opposite hand and soften around your neck, eyes, jaw, neck, head, and mind.

4. You can hold this pose for as long as you feel comfortable. Take your time coming out of this pose if you have any history of low blood pressure.

TIP: To enhance the stress and anxiety-relieving effect of this pose, visualize your worries melting away from the top of your head and absorbed by the ground around you literarily.

Child's Pose (Balasana)

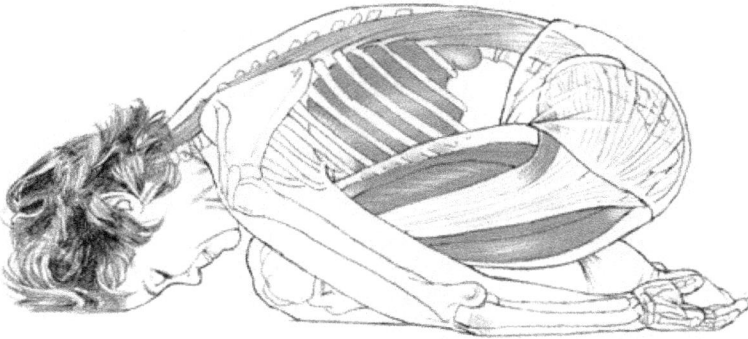

Whenever you feel frazzled, you tend to put lots of pressure on your adrenal glands, which can always lead to burnout and increased stress. The child pose is quite soothing for adrenals and therefore, doing the child pose often can give you the effect of a bubble bath, giant hug, and a bowl of soup all in one package.

Steps to the Balasana pose:

1. Stay down on your hands and knees, and then take the sit-bones back over your heels and your hands out in front of you. Fold your torso forward in a very slow move until you can feel your eyebrow touching the center of your yoga mat.

2. You can keep your knees together or separate them a bit wider than your hips; whichever way, make sure your toes are touching.

3. Keep your arms traditionally resting back alongside your body with your palms held up, but make sure you can stack your forearms and hands and still rest your head there if you think that is more preferable.

4. If your butt or hips are not touching your heels, you can simply place a cushion in between to help you let go and relax more. Hold the pose for 10 breaths or more and let go as much as possible with each exhalation.

5. Visualize a soothing color at the eyebrow center such as lilac, gold, or blue. Imagine that color flowing in and out of each breath you take, calming and soothing your mind as you go.

The Thunderbolt Pose (Vajrasana)

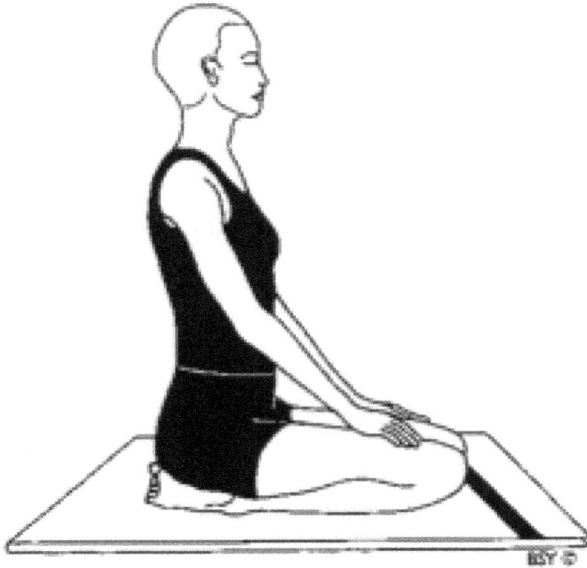

The thunderbolt has a powerful soothing effect on your mind and body. If your high stress levels and tension give you digestive problems, this pose will help you relieve it.

Steps to the Thunderbolt pose:

1. Get on your knees, and from the kneeling position, sit back on your heels. You can keep a cushion between your sit-bones and your feet if you feel comfortable enough with that.

2. Maintain a straight spine, and feel your crown draw up towards the ceiling.

3. Cross your hands in front of your chest and cup your palms at your underarms. Keep your thumps up in front of you.

4. Connect with your breath as you notice how fast your mind starts calming and slowing down. Hold the pose for about 10 minutes and imagine yourself releasing stress and tension with every breath you exhale.

5. If you are not comfortable sitting on your knees for that long, you can cross your legs.

TIP: Do this before bedtime every night to help you enjoy better sleep at night.

Reclined Bound Angle Pose (Supta Baddha Konasana)

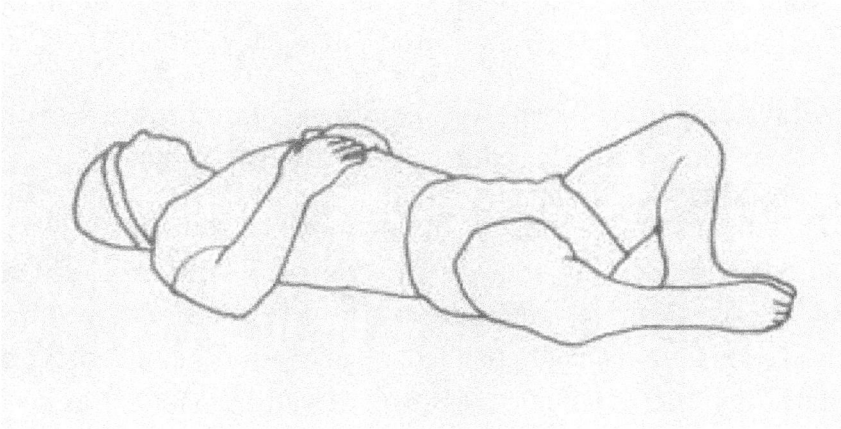

This pose will make you feel like you have embarked on a mini stress-relieving vacation. It can help you open through the inner thighs, hips, and groin; all of the places where you can hold stress and tension. The floor beneath you will give you the support you need to surrender to the moment and practice the calming art of letting go.

Steps to the Reclined Bound Angle pose:

1. Lie on your back in a Savasana pose. Bring the soles of your feet together, with your knees out to the side. If one or both of your knees are a bit far from the floor, you can use yoga blocks, folded blankets, or bolsters underneath them in order to ensure the pose is more soothing.

2. As for your arms, you can lift them overhead and take each one of your elbows with your opposite hands, or you

can keep them resting on the floor alongside your torso. Alternatively, you can place one hand on your belly and the other on your heart center to create a soothing connection within you.

3. Stay for as long as you feel comfortable and move slowly when you are finally ready to come out of this pose.

TIP: This gives you a great opportunity to reinforce a very positive and calming message to yourself. You can add a mantra or positive affirmation to every inhalation and exhalation such as "I choose to be relaxed and calm" as you inhale and "I let go of all stress, worries and anxieties" as you exhale.

The Corpse Pose (Savasana)

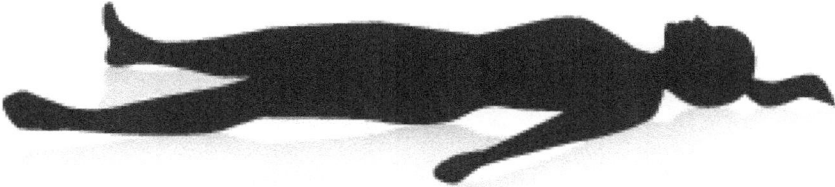

This is the easiest yoga pose to do physically, but many yogis consider it the most difficult for the mind to master.

Steps to the Corpse pose:

1. Lie still on your yoga mat, with your arms placed on both sides, palms facing upwards, legs relaxed, and your feet turning towards the side of your mat.

2. If you feel tension at your lower back, you can support it with a pillow.

3. Slowly close the eyes and consciously release any tension in your face

4. Practice deep breathing until you are very relaxed. Stay in the moment and refuse to dwell on any invading thoughts

We mentioned deep breathing casually in some of the yoga poses. Let us now see what deep breathing is all about and how you can harness its benefits as one of the key techniques for combating stress and its attendant problems in your day-to-day life.

2ⁿᵈ Technique: Deep breathing For Stress and Anxiety Relief

When done accurately, deep breathing can bring instant relief to your stress, anxiety, and depression thanks to its very calming effects.

Let us begin by learning how to breathe properly:

How to Breath (Deep Breathe) Properly

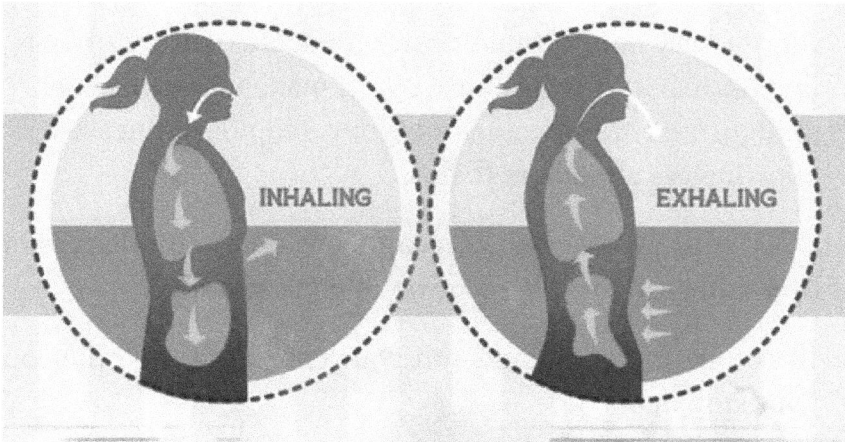

As strange as it may sound, most people do not know how to breathe properly. Natural breathing should involve the whole of your diaphragm and a large muscle in your abdomen.

Your belly should expand whenever you breathe in and fall as you breathe out. We call this diaphragmatic breathing. People forget the right way to breathe overtime, which is the major cause of the stress and anxiety because it causes shallow breaths that we take with using our shoulders and chest alone.

Well, even if you have been doing the breathing thing the wrong way for so long, it is never too late to unlearn the wrong breathing pattern in order to relearn the right pattern as a way of keeping yourself protected from stress.

Here are some simple steps you can take to improve your breathing:

1. Find a very comfortable position such as sitting or lying on your back. If you choose to sit, make sure your back is straight and the tensions on your shoulders released by allowing the shoulders to drop.

2. Close your eyes so that you can focus on the mechanics of breathing rather than focus on outside stimuli.

3. Place one of your hands on your chest and the other on your stomach

4. Take in a few deep breaths. Take note of how your belly rises with each inhalation and falls with each exhalation.

5. Keep practicing deep breathing until you can associate in breaths and out breaths with the rising and falling of your belly.

Basic Deep Breathing Tips You Will Find Useful

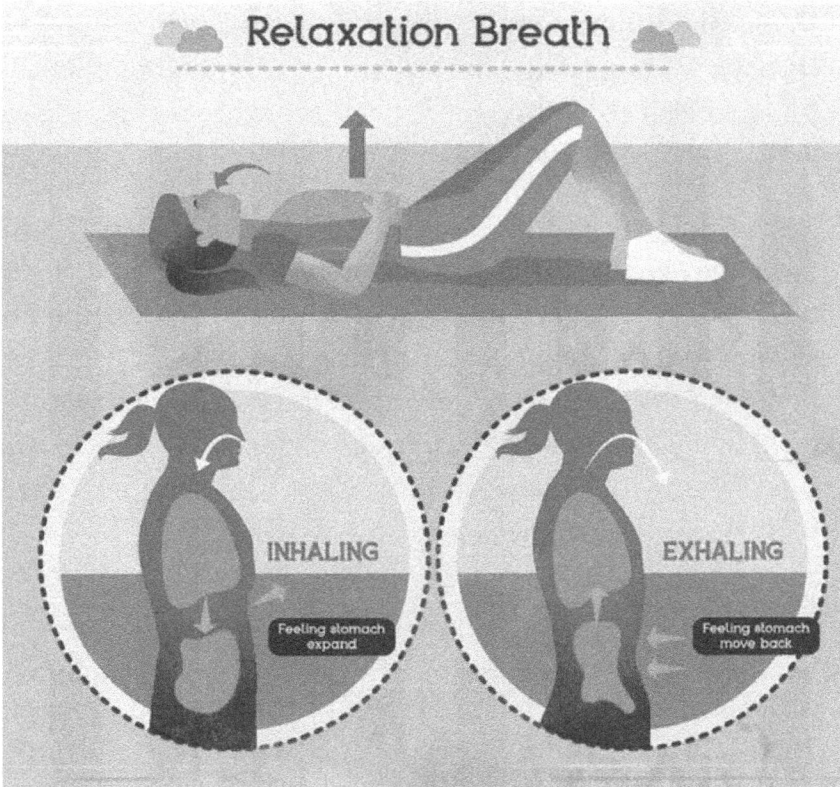

1. Relearning how to breathe can take some time. However, this art will become easier with frequent practices. You can take out some time every day to engage in deep breathing exercises. The good thing about practicing deep breathing to beat stress is that you can do it almost anywhere and at any time of the day.

2. Try practicing whenever you feel calm and relaxed. This will make taking in deep breaths easier for you.

3. If you find it hard to take in deep breaths, try breathing in through your nostrils and exhaling through your mouth. You can also count to 5 mentally whenever you breathe in and out.

4. With time, you can tell how long you practice before you feel relieved from stress, tension, or anxiety. You can set time limits as a beginner, like, 3 minutes per session, several times a day. Always remember that it is more beneficial to practice several short breaths a day than to engage in a single long deep breathing episode. Practicing more often will help incorporate deep breathing into your daily life and schedules.

Let us now talk about the progressive muscle relaxation technique:

3rd Technique: Progressive Muscle Relaxation Anxiety, Depression, Stress & Tension Relief

This is a two-step process where you systematically tense and relax different group of muscles in your body. If practiced regularly, you become intimately familiar with that muscle tension that tells you your body needs rest. This familiarity will teach you to react swiftly and accordingly to the very first signs of muscular tension that accompany stress.

Your body's relaxation goes hand-in-hand with your mind relaxation—just in case you start wondering how relaxing your muscles helps you deal with anxiety and depression. For enhanced results, you can combine progressive muscle relaxation with other relaxation techniques such as deep breathing.

How to Practice Progressive Muscle Relaxation

If you have ever had any issues of back problems, muscle spasms, or other such serious injuries that may have led to tension in your muscles, you may need to consult your doctor before you embark on this muscle relaxation technique.

Here is what to do:

1. The idea is to begin at your feet and work your way up to your facial muscles (or the other way round).

2. Loosen your clothes, take your shoes off, and get as comfortable as possible.

3. Take a couple of minutes to practice deep breathing

4. When you are set, simply shift all attention to your right foot. Take some minutes to understand how the foot feels at that moment.

5. Slowly tense the muscles of the right foot, squeezing those muscles as tightly as possible. You can hold and count from 1-10.

6. Relax your foot before focusing on the tension as it flows away from your right foot and note how the foot feels as it becomes loose and limp.

7. Stay in this state of relaxation briefly and breathe in slowly, but deeply.

8. Shift all attention to your left foot and follow the same process you used for the right foot.

9. Slowly move up through the body, where you contract as well as relax the various muscle groups while going up.

10. This will take some regular practices at first, but always make sure you never tense any other muscles save the ones you are focusing on at any point

Here is a good muscle relaxation sequence you can work with:

1. Right foot

2. Left foot

3. Right calf

4. Left calf

5. Hips and buttocks

6. Stomach

7. Chest

8. Back

9. Right arm and hand

10. Left arm and hand

11. Neck and shoulders

12. Face

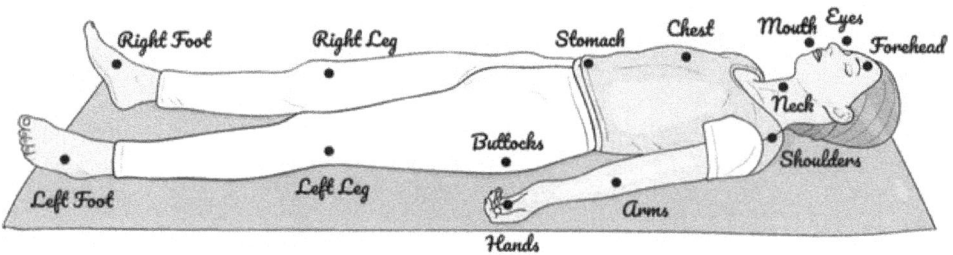

4th Technique: Body Scan Meditation for Stress and Anxiety Relief

The body scan meditation is a form of meditation that focuses your whole attention on different parts of the body. Just like the progressive muscle relaxation technique that we discussed earlier, you begin with the feet and then work all the way up to your facial muscles.

It differs from the progressive muscle relaxation in that in this instance, you do not need to tense your muscles. You simply focus on how each part feels, without judging the feeling as either positive or negative.

How to Practice Body Scan Meditation

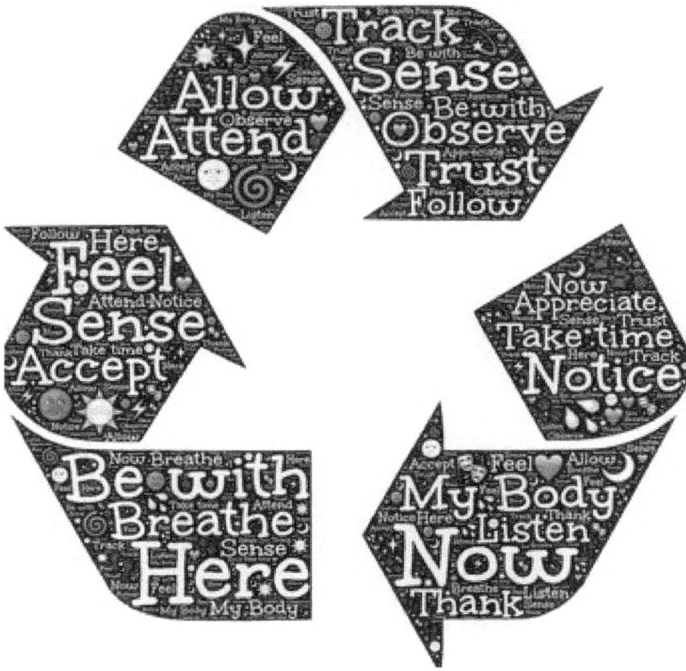

Here are steps to the muscle scan meditation:

1. Lie on your back and keep your arms relaxed at your sides without crossing your legs. You can leave your eyes open or closed.

2. Focus on your right toes. Take note of any sensation present in those toes even as you focus on your breathing. Imagine each of the deep breaths you take flowing to your toes. Maintain your focus on that area for 1-3 minutes.

3. Move that focus to the right sole. Become aware of the sensation on your right sole and imagine each breath you take flowing from the right sole. Maintain your focus for 1-3 minutes before moving it to your right ankle.

4. Move your focus to your calf, then the knee, followed by thigh, and then the hip and repeat the sequence for your left leg beginning with the toes and ending with the left hipbone. From there, you can then move to your torso, through your lower back abdomen, your upper back, your chest, and your shoulders. If you get to any part that gives you some pain and discomfort, pay closer attention and spend longer there until you sense the tension and pain drifting away.

5. Once done with your body scan, relax for some minutes— say 5-7 minutes—in stillness and silence, taking note of how your body feels. You can then slowly open your eyes and stretch if need be.

Now comes the chief of all relaxation techniques: the mindfulness meditation technique. Each one of the techniques we have mentioned thus far draws strength from this one.

5th Technique: Mindfulness Meditation

Mindfulness meditation is a relaxation technique that can help you switch your focus from past regrets and future worries to what is happening around you at any given moment. This allows you to engage fully in the present moment and helps you enjoy life as it happens, which is why it is highly effective for combating stress, anxiety and depression.

For ages, man has used meditations that cultivate mindfulness to reduce stress, anxiety, depression, and all other negative mood disorders. Some mindful meditation techniques help you focus on one single repetitive action such as deep breathing, a few mantras, positive self-talks/affirmations, or the flickering light of a candle.

The good thing about mindful meditation is that once it becomes a part of your daily life, you can easily translate mindfulness into your normal daily routines and do things with increased concentration and accuracy. Other activities you can do mindfully to further win the battle with stress, anxiety, and depression include mindful walking, dancing, workout, eating, bath, washing, home chores, etc.

Basic Mindfulness Meditation

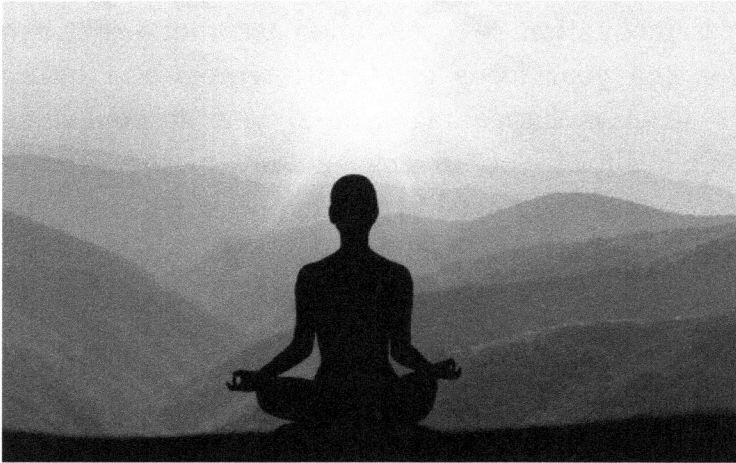

Here are the basic steps to mindful meditation:

1. Get yourself comfortably seated on a straight-back chair or sit cross-legged on the floor.

2. Choose one aspect of your breathing and focus on it such as the sound of air rushing in and out of your airways, the sensation of inhalation and exhalation, the rise and fall of your belly, etc.

3. The moment your concentration narrows, start widening your focus and become aware of every sound, thought, and sensation present.

4. Embrace and consider every sensation or thought without being judgmental. If you catch your thoughts straying at any point, simply bring it back to focus on that aspect of

your breathing you chose before widening your awareness once more.

You can get more from your mindful meditation sessions by incorporating two powerful relaxation tools: visualization and positive self-talks:

1: **Visualization**

You can incorporate visualization into your mindful meditation sessions. However, it can be a powerful tool for the treatment of stress, depression, and anxiety on its own.

Visualization, also called guided imagery, involves imagining a scene that makes you feel at peace and free from every trace of anxiety and tension. Choose whatever you find most appealing and peaceful such as your favorite childhood spot, a quiet forest path, a tropical beach, a riverbank, an ocean view, etc.

You can practice visualization with the aid of listening aids such as soothing music, recordings that match your chosen setting, sound machine, or in silence. If you have chosen to visualize a beach, the sound of ocean waves will be ideal.

Steps to visualization:

1. Close your eyes and imagine a peaceful setting.

2. Picture the setting as vividly as possible: see, hear, smell, taste, and feel everything in that setting. Visualization works best when all sensory details involving all the senses are incorporated. If you are imagining a dock for instance, see the sun set over the water, hear the birds sing, smell the pine trees, feel the coldness of the water as it overflows the riverbank and touches your bare feet, taste the clean, and fresh air.

3. Imagine your worries, anxieties, and fears drifting away as you explore your serene environment and enjoy its restfulness.

4. When done, calmly open your eyes and return to the present. You will be amazed at how calm and relaxed you will feel.

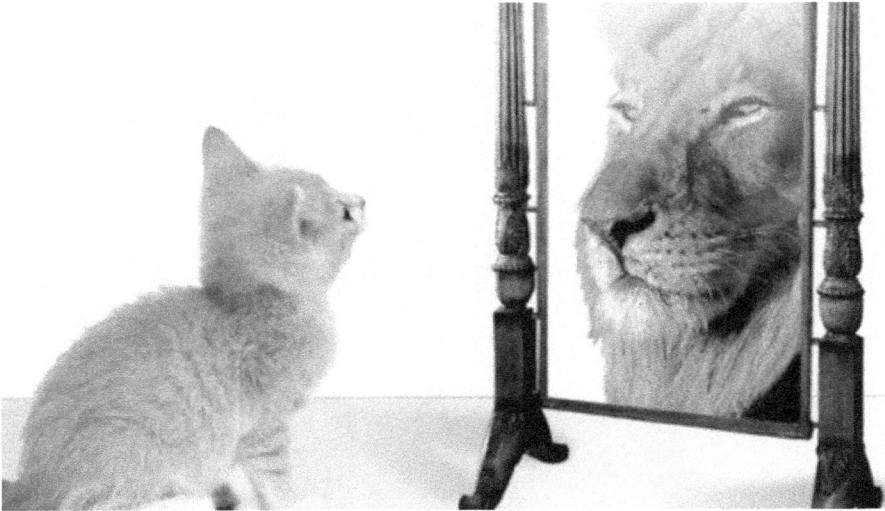

2: Positive Self-Talk

If your 5-year old son were to tell you he is nervous about going to school the next day, what would be your response? You are not likely to tell the child he is being dumb and behaving like a sissy. You would probably want to find out if the child is a victim of is bullying or why he feels nervous about going to school.

We seem so good at helping people we care about deal with stress and stressors in their lives, and yet find it difficult to handle our own stress issues.

In the same way you would reassure your child there is nothing to be anxious about, you should learn to use some positive self-talks on yourself whenever you feel nervous, stressed out, or tensed up.

Here are some examples of phrases you can coin into positive self-talks and incorporate into your mindful meditation session to help you feel more comfortable and relaxed when there are reasons for nerves to become ruffled:

1. "I have been through worse issues in the past; I will get through this as well."

2. "This feeling shall pass."

3. "There is no reason to panic or feel anxious right now."

4. "All is well with me and all that are mine."

5. "I feel safe right now."

6. "I have the power to make myself calm despite the anxiety I feel right now."

7. "I can feel my taut muscles relaxing and my heart rate slowing down."

NOTE: These meditations become more successful when done in very serene and private environments where the chances of interruption are minimal. Also, make sure you experiment with different sitting positions to know one you are most comfortable with. Avoid lying down as it may make you sleep off during meditation.

Final Tips to Help You Live a Stress-Free Life

The following tips build on what we have learnt thus far:

Know your stressors and avoid them

You should be able to identify what triggers your stress and avoid such triggers. Know friends whose company makes you feel terrible about life and stay away from them. Know places you visit and come home in very low spirits and avoid such places. Know habits that make you sick and negative such as gluttony, drunkenness, late night movies, social media addictions and avoid them.

Embrace minimalism

Learn to be satisfied with little. Reduce your number of friends, your daily tasks, and activities, de-clutter your home, get rid of useless clutter, and keep only things you really need. This will reduce your workload, increase the amount of free time with which you get practice the 5 key techniques discussed in this guide, and give you more peace of mind with increased productivity.

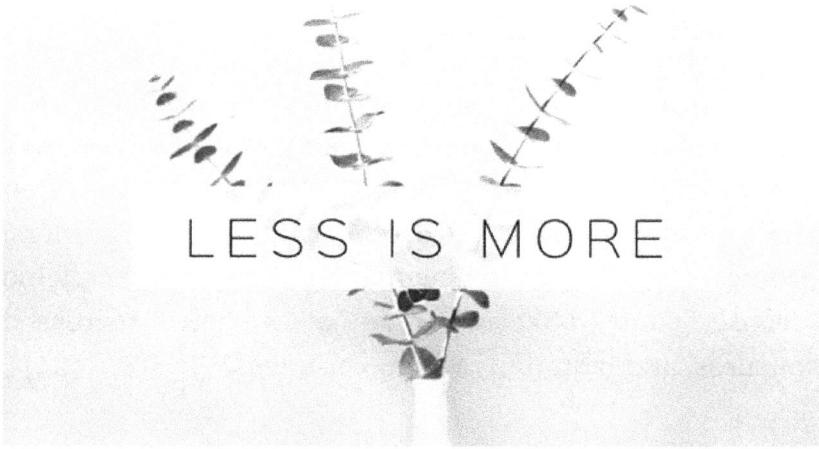

LESS IS MORE

Pay attention to your diet

It may surprise you to know that what you eat and drink most times affect your mood more than you would have ever thought possible. Foods containing alcohol and caffeine often associate with worsened cases of anxiety disorders. According to studies, even the slightest amount of caffeine can cause panic attacks, bouts of anxiety, increased nervousness, and irritability when consumed.

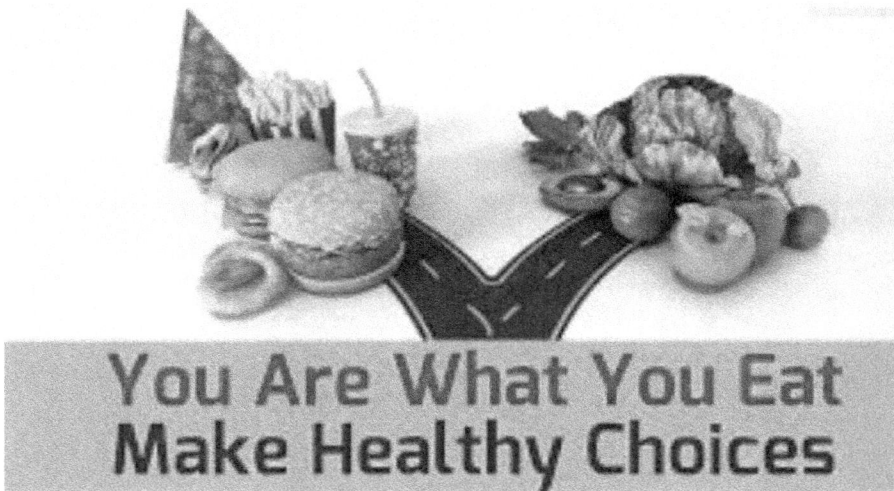

You Are What You Eat
Make Healthy Choices

Get adequate sleep

Almost all of us feel a bit crabby after what we can only call a rough night's sleep. Most people dealing with emotional disorders have disrupted sleep to wrestle with every night. Sometimes it is not easy to tell which one started before the other between the high stress levels and poor sleep habits. According to a study conducted by researchers at

Pennsylvania University, losing a few hours of sleep can increase your stress, exhaustion, anger, and sadness levels.

Stay Fit and active

We all know how important daily physical exercises are to our body and overall health. Research studies conducted in the last couple of decades suggest that exercise is far more effective than medications.

Maintaining a healthy exercise routine minimizes stress, enhance self-esteem, increase your energy levels, and enhance your mood. During these physical exercises, your body releases chemicals known as endorphins, chemicals that can interact with receptors in your brain to cause those feelings of euphoria and conceal physical pains.

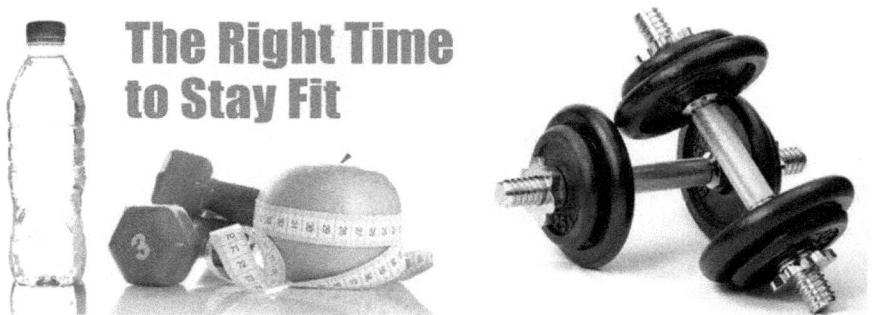

Build better connections

You need to make new friends who can bring new excitement and sunshine into your life. The more fun you have, the less time you will have to worry about a future you cannot influence and regret past mistakes you cannot correct. Stay away from toxic people and learn to say no to people and activities that eat up your productive time and keep you disorganized.

Engage yourself meaningfully

Find a new cause or hobby that will challenge, excite, and keep you occupied. You can volunteer for a nonprofit and engage in more outdoor campaigns to let in some more sunshine into your life and bring in some positive value to the world you live in.

Conclusion

We have come to the end of the book. Thank you for reading and congratulations for reading until the end.

It may not be entirely possible to live without stress, anxiety or depression as no one can accurately predict tomorrow. However, with the techniques and tips outlined in this book, you can manage your stress effectively and keep them as low as possible at all times.

If you found the book valuable, can you recommend it to others? One way to do that is to post a review on Amazon.

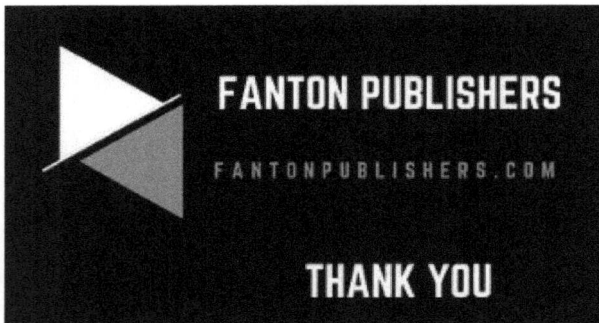

FANTON PUBLISHERS

FANTONPUBLISHERS.COM

THANK YOU

Do You Like My Book & Approach To Publishing?

If you like my writing and style and would love the ease of learning literally everything you can get your hands on from Fantonpublishers.com, I'd really need you to do me either of the following favors.

1: First, I'd Love It If You Leave a Review of This Book on Amazon.

2: Check Out My Emotional Mastery Books

Note: This list may not represent all my Keto diet books. You can check the full list by visiting my author page.

Emotional Intelligence: The Mindfulness Guide To Mastering Your Emotions, Getting Ahead And Improving Your Life

Stress: The Psychology of Managing Pressure: Practical Strategies to turn Pressure into Positive Energy (5 Key Stress Techniques for Stress, Anxiety, and Depression Relief)

Failure Is Not The END: It Is An Emotional Gym: Complete Workout Plan On How To Build Your Emotional Muscle And Burning Down Anxiety To Become Emotionally Stronger, More Confident and Less Reactive

[Subconscious Mind: Tame, Reprogram & Control Your Subconscious Mind To Transform Your Life](#)

[Body Language: Master Body Language: A Practical Guide to Understanding Nonverbal Communication and Improving Your Relationships](#)

[Shame and Guilt: Overcoming Shame and Guilt: Step By Step Guide On How to Overcome Shame and Guilt for Good](#)

[Anger Management: A Simple Guide on How to Deal with Anger](#)

Get updates when we publish any book that will help you master your emotions: http://bit.ly/2fantonpubpersonaldevl

To get a list of all my other books, please fantonwriters.com, my author central or let me send you the list by requesting them below: http://bit.ly/2fantonpubnewbooks

3: Grab Some Freebies On Your Way Out; Giving Is Receiving, Right?

I gave you a complimentary book at the start of the book. If you are still interested, grab it here.

[5 Pillar Life Transformation Checklist](#): http://bit.ly/2fantonfreebie

PSS: Let Me Also Help You Save Some Money!

If you are a heavy reader, have you considered subscribing to Kindle Unlimited? You can read this and millions of other books for just $9.99 a month)! You can check it out by searching for Kindle Unlimited on Amazon!

www.ingramcontent.com/pod-product-compliance
Lightning Source LLC
Chambersburg PA
CBHW031135020426
42333CB00012B/382